grown-up
&
gorgeous

in your 50s

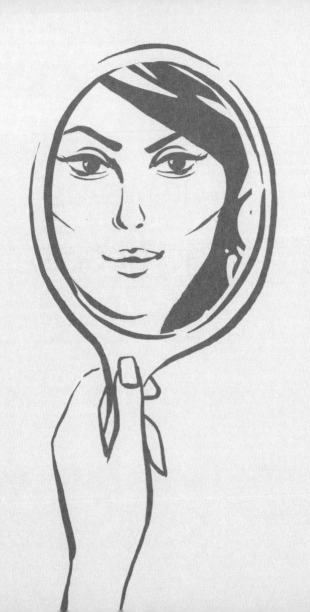

grown-up
&
gorgeous
in your 50s

Pamela Robson

EBURY
PRESS

Acknowledgements: Dr Mary Dingley, President of the Australasian Society of Cosmetic Physicians; Tanja Mrnjaus, ID Couture, Melbourne, Sydney and Brisbane; Dr Shane Rea, Barshop Institute for Longevity and Aging Studies, University of Texas; Ken Gordon & Toni Adams, Musculo-Skeletal Clinic, Spring Hill, Queensland; Dr Cathy Gaulton, Pacific Cosmetic Surgery, Brisbane, Queensland; Jean Hailes Foundation; Wellesley College Biology Department, Maryland; American Academy of Peridontology

Contents

*f*ifty-something? You're in your prime. The kids are off your hands – well, almost. You know what you want out of life – well, almost. You're at the top of your career and enjoying it – mostly. You have a wisdom born of experience. And you're still looking pretty hot.

For the first time in your life you feel in control. You aspire to make the best of yourself and your future. You want to make the most of your mature beauty. Birthdays may be inevitable, but looking older than you feel doesn't have to be. With knowledge and lifestyle changes, you can actually feel and look better at 50 than you did at 30. It's an empowering evolution.

This is the decade to take stock, and to set in place good practices and goals that will carry you, happy and healthy, into your 60s.

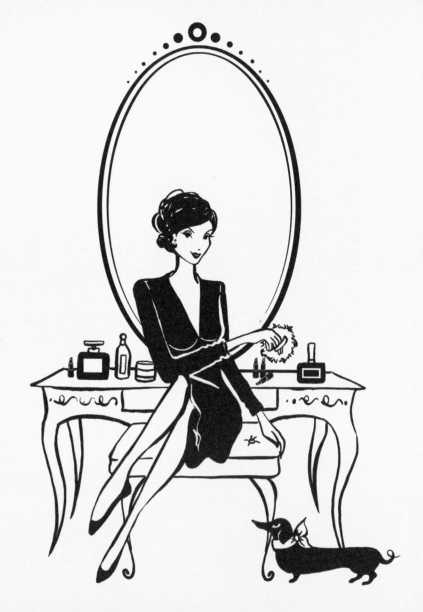

Beauty

Now that you're in your 50s, you're finally comfortable in your own skin. No more comparing yourself to others, you've learned to relax and have realistic expectations about your face and hair. You don't want to look younger, or like someone else – it's about looking as great as you can for your age.

Ageing is amazing

Your skin doesn't lie. Certainly, genetics play a big role in how you look now, but the way you treated your skin (from the inside and on the outside) in the past will also determine how you're ageing. Your lifestyle choices will have an impact, but some skin changes during this decade are beyond your control: the skin renewal process will be slowing down, and hormonal changes will also have an effect. There are, however, more and more ways to minimise the damage! Skincare, make-up and your crowning glory are fantastic weapons.

Your 50-something face

The three Ss

Sun, smoking and (lack of) sleep ... Nothing will make you look older than your years than indulging in these beauty crimes! Prevention is better than the cure.

Sun-tanning

The fastest way to look old is to lie in the sun. Sun damage is now considered *the* most important factor in skin ageing, accounting for 90 per cent of the damage you see. If you don't believe this, just compare the skin on your hands with that on your bum! It's never too late to protect your skin, so start slathering on the SPF 30 religiously.

Smoking

The next biggest age accelerator is smoking, which affects your skin at a cellular level. In response to the toxins in tobacco, your body forms 'free radicals' – unstable molecules that damage cell DNA. Smoking also hardens

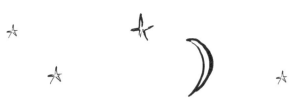

the arteries, restricting blood flow and preventing oxygen getting to the skin. It increases production of an enzyme that breaks down the supply of the skin's main building material, collagen. It also reduces the body's stores of vitamin A and blocks absorption of vitamin C – both vital for healthy skin. And we haven't even mentioned those nasty smokers' lines that radiate from a constantly puckered mouth …

Sleeping

It's not called beauty sleep for nothing! When you're asleep, your skin cells go into overtime, renewing themselves and repairing damage. Research shows that between 10pm and 2am your skin cells are most actively rejuvenating themselves.

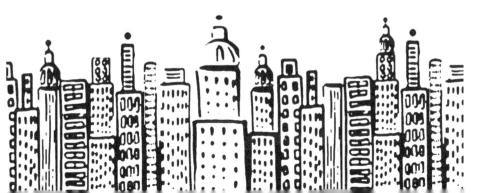

Skincare

No amount of make-up will make up for a non-existent skincare routine! Many factors determine how your skin will look and feel, day to day (think genetics, diet, the weather, stress), but if you follow a sensible skincare regimen that's tailored to your needs you'll notice a huge difference in your complexion. Once, the golden rule of skincare was: cleanse, tone and moisturise. Now it's: cleanse, exfoliate, moisturise and protect, and protect, protect, protect.

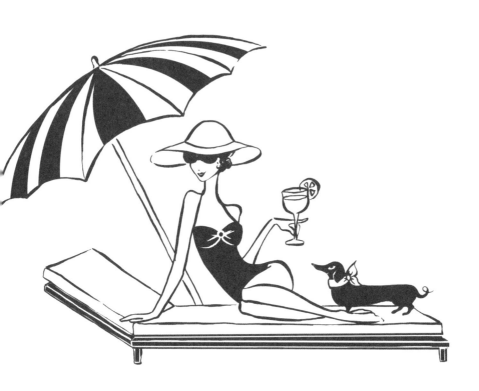

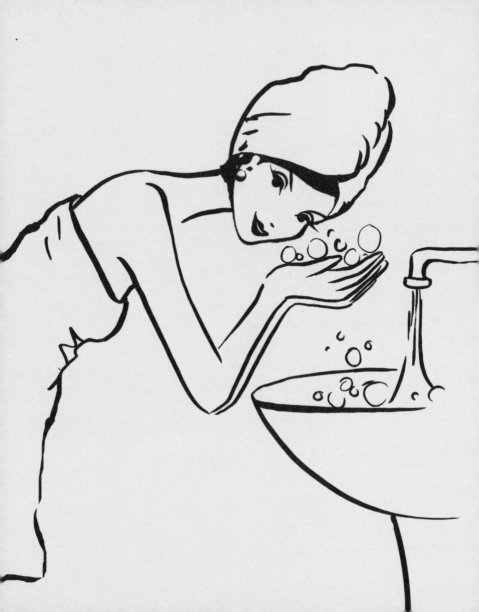

Cleanse

Remove dead skin cells, dirt and pollutants with a cleanser (preferably twice a day). Choose a cream or oil-based cleanser if your skin feels dry; foaming gel-based cleansers are great if your skin feels oily. Never use body soap on your face. Today's cleansers don't require toner afterwards, and many dermatologists consider them to be drying, but if you like the feel of a toner, pick one without alcohol in it.

Exfoliate

Exfoliators are designed to help remove dead skin cells, which becomes very important as the cell renewal process slows down with age. Exfoliation removes the top, dry layer of skin cells, stimulates cell turnover and revs up collagen production. Cosmetic procedures such as chemical peels and dermabrasion are simply more aggressive forms of exfoliation. Every three days or so, use a gentle facial exfoliant *after* you've cleansed.

Moisturise

Nothing will make you look fresher than well-hydrated skin. Tackling dehydration from the inside out is essential, so drink plenty of water each day. Externally, moisturisers will provide an immediate 'plumping' effect, while helping your skin to retain surface moisture. Pick a lightweight lotion for daytime; a richer one for night (or whenever your skin feels drier, such as during winter). Be careful when choosing expensive formulas with complicated claims (such as active vitamin C creams); some products work, others don't. Seek professional advice.

drink plenty of water each day

Protect

The easiest way to cover up is to choose foundation and moisturiser containing a broad-spectrum (UVA and UVB) sunscreen – SPF 30 is ideal for our Australian climate. While SPF is a measure of protection against UVB, the rays that cause sunburn, higher SPF sunscreens usually offer greater protection against UVA, the rays most responsible for premature ageing. It is also claimed that a sunscreen with built-in antioxidants offers even more protection.

Tough but true!

Having a 30-year-old face and 80-year-old cleavage is not a good look. Please protect your décolletage (and hands) with sunblock. Sun-damage-minimising techniques such as exfoliation, peels, laser and dermabrasion don't work as well on these areas as they don't have the same number of sebaceous glands as the face, which means they don't heal as quickly.

Make-up

As we age, our faces demand different make-up and application techniques. Heavy products can make us look a decade older than we really are. Repeat every morning as you face the mirror: I will be pretty and fresh, not severe and old. The goal is to look natural – just as you are, but better.

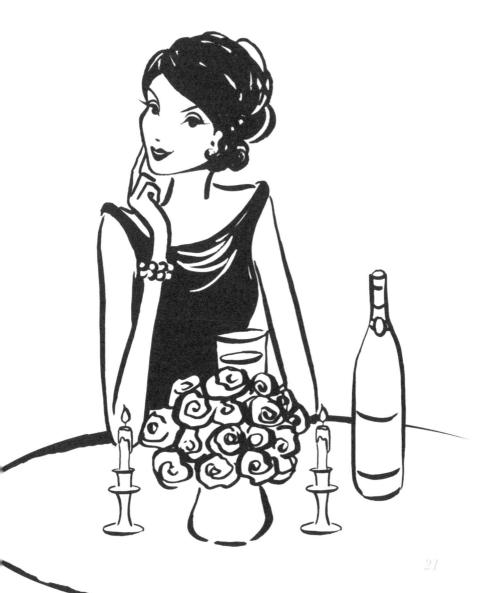

The perfect make-up kit

Here's what you should have in your make-up repertoire:

A light-reflecting foundation

★

Concealer

★

Mascara

★

Eyeshadow
(neutral, natural light, medium and dark shades)

★

Lip gloss

★

Lipstick

★

Blush and bronzer

A note on blush and bronzer...

Don't underestimate what a dash of colour can do for your looks! Not just for the under-30s, well-placed blush will make you look pretty, youthful and give you that just-exercised glow (to choose the hue, pick one that most closely matches your natural post-workout flush). Powder blushes are easiest to work with, while cream blush adds a dewy touch. Approach bronzer in a similar manner: for a sun-kissed glow, swirl a little onto the apples of your cheeks, and where the sun would naturally tan your face (a dash across your brow bone, nose, chin and your collarbones). Avoid orange-toned, frosted formulas and pick brown-based bronzers in a shade that's only slightly darker than your complexion.

Back to base

A beautiful complexion is your biggest asset;
it's an accessory in itself. Beauty trends come
and go, but flawless skin is in every season, every
year – we're talking dewy, fresh and natural.
Yet it's easy to get stuck in a time warp, wearing
foundation that looks like, well, foundation. It's
almost a century since Max Factor and Elizabeth
Arden took pancake make-up from the (silent)
silver screen and sold it to shopgirls. Today a
cakey, powdery base can make even the prettiest
woman look like a drag queen – and certainly far
older than her age. The solution? Take advantage
of technology, and look for foundation that
contains light-reflecting properties. Trial different
brands at the department store beauty counters.
Bases that promise to make your skin 'dewy' or
'luminous' contain particles that bounce light off,
creating the illusion of a fresh, smooth surface.

Your skin becomes drier with age and your make-up must allow for this. Rather than using a regular foundation (which can be too matte), consider tinted moisturisers or moisturising foundations. There are products out there that multi-task beautifully: moisturiser, light foundation or face tint, and sunscreen, all in one! There is a whole industry competing for the older woman's complexion – which means there are many new products containing anti-ageing and light-reflecting ingredients.

Here's an idea

Apply a creamy concealer that's about two shades lighter than your skin tone on dark eye circles. This instantly makes you look more rested and youthful.

Making eyes

Once the skin on your eyelids starts to become crepey (or if the skin on the upper lids has started to droop, or if your eyes are losing that definition they used to have), there is a whole new set of make-up rules to learn. For example, multi-tiered colours of eyeshadow are too complicated for older lids. Instead, use two neutral shades and blend them so they look natural.

EXPERT TIP

A dab of concealer at the inner eye corners, blended well, will really make you look bright, fresh and awake.

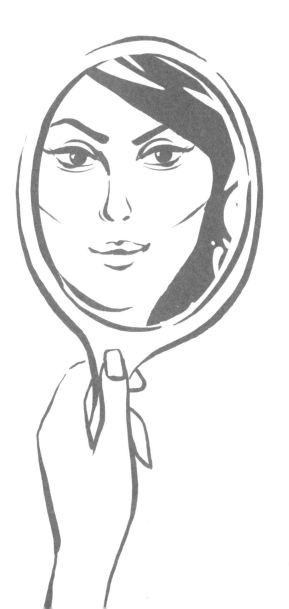

Crepey lids: Resist the temptation of shimmery or bright colours. They magnify imperfections. Stay away from dry, powdery products that can exaggerate crepey skin; likewise, be careful of greasy creams that can 'pond' in folds. Pick a soft, matte cream in natural shades – and lightly press face powder over your lids with a puff before you apply shadow, to create a smoother-looking surface.

The eye issues

Loss of definition: Smudge a soft wisp of eye pencil along your upper lashline, in flattering natural shades. Try to get it as close to the lashes as possible, starting from the inner eye and working out. A couple of coats of very black mascara will also work wonders.

Droopy lids: 'Bedroom' eyes can be very sexy – just look at actresses Ellen Barkin and Charlotte Rampling! But if the droop has gone beyond sexy and entered the realm of plain old tired, don't resort to surgery just yet – have your eyebrows shaped by a professional (more on this on page 31) and define your upper lashes with mascara.

Dark circles: The correct concealer will really help with this common problem, as will avoiding liner and mascara on the lower lashes. A dusting of pastel pink blush on the apples of your cheeks is a clever way to distract attention from the dark circles.

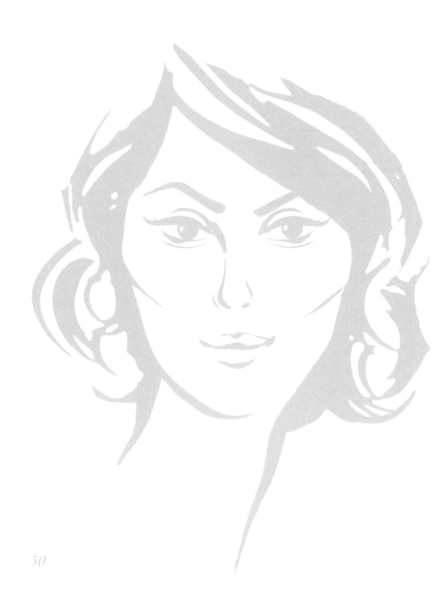

Brows

The carefree unruly brows that looked charming in our 20s look downright untidy in our 50s. Worse still, they can appear quite masculine. As with everything else on an ageing face, brows need more maintenance as the years pass. Fortunately, brows are finally being given the credit they deserve for the role they play in framing the face. Brow stylists and brow bars are no longer a rare commodity and this means there's plenty of expert help for those who don't want to venture into brow shaping and tinting on a DIY basis. If you've never had your brows done professionally, you are in for a treat. You'll be amazed at the difference a set of shaped and tinted brows can make (some women swear it's as good as a facelift!). This is one beauty treatment that is value for money.

Want to DIY?

Have an initial session with a professional brow stylist. Observe their techniques (usually waxing, plucking and tinting) and take note of where they place the arch.

When shaping your own brows, get comfortable in front of a regular mirror (not magnifying) and make sure the lighting is good, and natural.

Pluck two hairs at a time, from under the arch – checking your handiwork as you go.

Here's an idea

Tattooing can be a good option for brows that can't be coaxed into shape through the usual means. A good cosmetic tattoo artist can create a new brow line, and, with the wayward hairs waxed out, it can make a big difference. Again, do your homework and only go to a practitioner who comes recommended for their ability to create natural-looking brows. Ask them to start with a colour that's closest to your natural shade – you can have the colour deepened over time.

Update your look instantly: buff up your brows

Grooming your brows immediately frames your face, balances features and makes your eyes brighter. Invest in a brow kit (several make-up brands carry one containing brow powder, brush and wax), then, to create a lovely, lasting shape, fill in sparse arches with powder using a mini angle brush, and finish with a coat of clear wax.

Lips

Unless you are one of those rare women blessed with luscious lips that have stayed that way throughout the decades, there is a fundamental rule that must be obeyed as you age: ditch the super-dark lipstick. Even if you've worn nothing but deep reds for as long as you can remember, go straight to your nearest department store and work your way through the lighter colours. As we age our lips lose collagen and they thin. The darker the lipstick colour, the thinner your lips will look. Just think about it. Why do you wear black pants? Worse still, there is nothing less attractive than seeing dark lipstick 'bleeding' into the lines around the mouth!

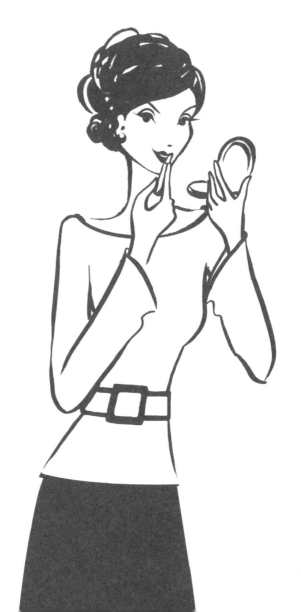

The lip issues

Thin lips: By all means define your lips with a liner, but it's best to use the same colour as your lipstick or just a shade darker. Choose shiny gloss and creamy lipsticks to give the illusion of fullness. Never line outside your lips, and don't waste money on products that claim to temporarily plump your lips – they can irritate your skin.

Loss of definition: As we age we lose lip definition, and if you've been quite minimalist in your make-up approach, you may find you now need a lip liner and lipstick. Again, don't line outside the mouth, and if you can still see the pencil after you've filled in your pout with lippie, blend the line with a lip brush to soften the look.

Lines around the mouth: Smoking is one of the main causes of these lines, as is sun damage and genetics. Prescription-based retinoid creams will help lessen the lines. Before applying lip colour, plump your pout with a hydrating balm (an eye cream will also work). Experts suggest lining and filling in your lips with a lip pencil, then apply lippie and top it off with a little gloss.

Loss of colour: Toss out your beige or brown lippie (they'll only emphasise the problem) in favour of vibrant cherry, berry, rose or apricot hues. A lip stain is a pretty way to add colour: make your own by mixing lip pencil and lip balm directly on your lips, and blending with your finger.

The classic red pout can be yours! It's important to know the shade that suits you. Women with 'cool' undertones to their skin should wear blue-based reds, while orange-brown shades look lovely on 'warm' skin.
TIP: if the veins on the inside of your arm look blue, your skin tone is cool; if they look green, it's warm.

Red lips at ANY age

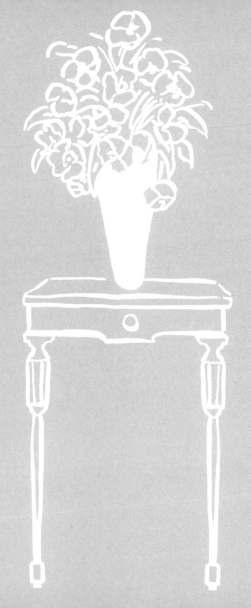

By your 50s, you've probably tried many a hairstyle and have come to some understanding about what works with your hair type and lifestyle. Whatever your natural hair colour, it's likely that grey hair has become quite noticeable, and your locks will have also become more brittle. But don't give up the battle and turn to the blue rinse! In your 50s, your hair really can be your crowning glory. So, how to stay modern, without having to be 'trendy'? You'll need to approach hair care, style and colour . . .

Your crowning glory

Be gentle

We're talking shampoo, conditioner and an intensive weekly treatment (if your hair is very dry, damaged or you use heat styling tools often). Choose gentle, moisturising formulas, and don't over-wash or over-condition your hair. Hair should squeak when you rinse the shampoo out, and conditioner should only be applied to the ends.

Gloss your locks

A gleaming, polished style will take years off your look. To re-create that salon shine, invest in a conditioning, glossing spray. Lightly spritz it over dry hair for a pick-me-up that flatters every shade – even grey.

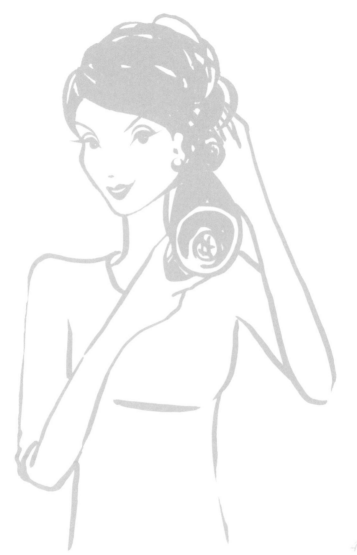

Let's be honest. The last time perfectly coiffed hair was fashionable was the 1960s, when hairspray was all the rage. It followed on from the stiff French pleat of the 1950s (think Hitchcock's blondes), the permed look of the war years and the lacquered wave of the 1920s Flappers. Today, hair that doesn't move screams 'old lady'. Your 50s is a time when less is definitely more – so it's important you find the perfect, simple cut. Hair should be casual, and look natural and healthy. So talk to your hairdresser about a style that works with your hair type, is easy to re-create at home and requires very little styling product.

The perfect, simple cut?

Experts are almost unanimous on this. It's the layered bob. Or, if you want to go longer, a shoulder-length cut with layers that softly frame your face. The best wash-and-go cut is a short 'do with lots of texture.

On the fringe

A fringe can hide a multitude of un-Botoxed brow lines, but keep it soft and layered. Short, thick fringes are hard to pull off and can overwhelm your face.

keep it soft and layered

It's a long story

Once, it was said that after 30 a woman shouldn't have long hair. Well, that's another rule we've said goodbye to! If your face isn't too thin, go for it. Just remember that straggly, thin, unkempt hair doesn't ever look good, no matter what your age.

Chop, chop!

Hair colour becomes very important in your 50s: you're probably in 'limbo' – neither totally grey nor your original colour. Silvery grey hair can be very beautiful (keep it this way with a colour-correcting 'violet' shampoo to neutralise yellowness), but if you're just not ready for it, there's an art to colouring your locks. Subtle colour changes can be done at home, but more drastic changes should be left to the professionals. The more grey you have, the trickier it is to camouflage – your hairdresser will need to add lowlights and highlights; an all-over colour will be too harsh and will leave you with very obvious regrowth. Basically, the older you get the lighter you need to go, as there is nothing so ageing as severe, dark colour.

Your true colours

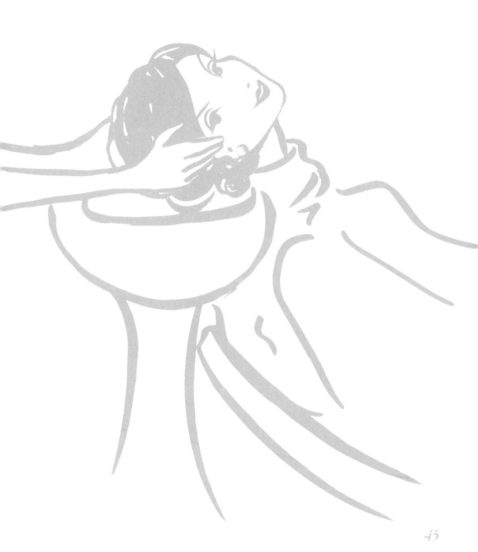

43

Highlights are simply made for women in their 50s – they'll lift and brighten your face in a subtle way, and they're universally flattering. A good hair colourist will strategically place them (and graduate the colour) to look natural – like you've been holidaying in the sun – *not* give you unnaturally uniform vertical stripes.

The light fantastic

EXPERT TIP

It's not only the hair on your head that goes grey as you get older; so does your facial hair. If you've made a subtle hair colour change, simply update your brow pencil or shadow. If you've drastically altered your colour, it's a good idea to have your brows dyed to match (your hair colourist should be able to do this for you).

Eek! Facial hair

It's one of those things that happens with menopause: eyebrows and lashes get sparser, while once-smooth areas such as the upper lip and the chin suddenly sprout the furry stuff. It's hormonal of course, and, as with everything else to do with ageing – completely unfair and indiscriminate. Some people grow an entire moustache and others don't see a single hair.

What to do?

When it comes to the face, it's worth spending time and money on professional hair removal. This means waxing at the beauty salon, or laser hair reduction. This zaps the hair at the follicle and permanently disables it. It can only work on the hair that is growing at the time, so you'll need several treatments. Still, once it's gone, it's gone! Both waxing and laser come with risks – they can burn. This means that you need to find a well-trained and experienced practitioner.

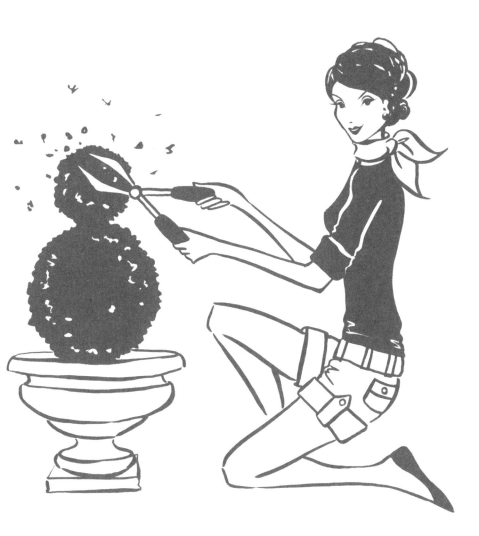

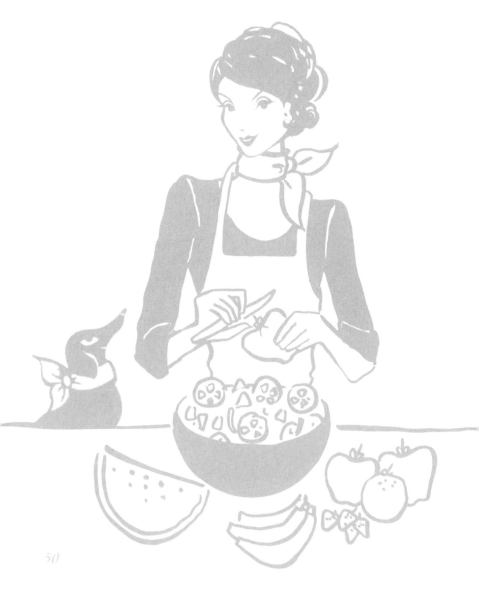

Cosmetic medicine

Is it really only 10 years since the word Botox entered
the beauty editors' vocabulary? Once the domain of
the rich and famous, it's now available to every woman.
We've come a long way in a short time. But you must
still approach it with caution. Cosmetic surgery is, like
everything else in your 50s, your own personal choice.
However, being 'grown-up and gorgeous' does not
automatically require a session with a surgeon. The
beauty and cosmetic medicine industries are constantly
creating new ways to hold off, or reverse, the years.
More and more, this involves non-surgical procedures.

The preventative approach

Thankfully, most of us are realistic about what cosmetic surgery can and can't do. These days, it's less about the surgery and more about the 'low-invasive' approach that can stave off the operating theatre. These are Botox, skin fillers and skin rejuvenation techniques. For example, the industry confidently predicts that women in their 30s using Botox to stop the onset of frown lines and other muscle-induced wrinkles are unlikely to be seeking surgery as early as their older sisters once did. And even if you didn't start having Botox until you were in your 40s, you've nevertheless positioned yourself well ahead of the game.

Take note!

Cosmetic medicine is an art as well as a science and the variation between practitioners is significant. Some have a natural talent and plenty of experience – others have neither, but are great salespeople. If you're interested in a treatment, please do your research.

THE AGEING FACE

You'll lose bone and muscle volume

You'll lose fat from your face – this especially
affects women who diet and exercise

Your cheek 'fat pads' descend, creating folds on either
side of your mouth, and blurring the jaw-line

The skin renewal process slows and skin becomes less elastic;
static lines and wrinkles develop

Photo-ageing – otherwise known as sun damage –
accumulates, creating coarser, crepey skin

Your upper eyelids will start to droop and bags
will appear under your eyes

Prominent vertical neck muscles may occur
if you have bad posture

The many uses of Botox

The way Botox is used is constantly being refined, and doctors today have a better understanding of where and how to inject for best results. Each practitioner has their favourite techniques and applications, and be mindful that some are more skilled at injecting than others.

Botox injections don't have to be overly painful.

Botox is known for its use on the upper half of the face: blocking the formation of frown lines across the forehead, crows' feet and bunny lines (those horizontal lines across the bridge of the nose). Botox can also be used to relax the downward pull of the muscles around the mouth, as a successful

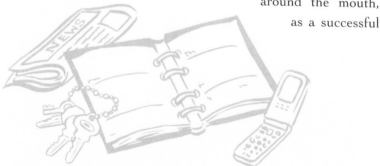

treatment for migraine and to reduce excessive armpit sweating. A promising new treatment is for prominent neck muscles, which occur as a result of bad posture. By injecting these muscles with Botox, they can be relaxed so that they don't stand out. The treatment can make a big difference, but many practitioners are wary of using Botox below the eye area.

EXPERT TIP

Like everything else in life, you get what you pay for. If a practitioner is offering you a cheap deal they may be using a more diluted concentration of Botox. This means it won't work as well and it won't last as long. A good treatment should last a couple of months. Many people find that as time goes on the effect seems to last longer and they need less frequent visits. Practitioners offering deals might also be new to the game and in need of more patients. If you go to a practitioner with L plates, you have to be prepared for the fact you might not get the best results. Avoid Botox parties (like Tupperware parties!) at all costs.

*There are as many types
of facelift as there are surgeons
performing them.*

The facelift is a very individual thing. It depends on the techniques used, the style preferred by the surgeon, and the quality of the original material (your face). There are deep facelifts where the surgeon lifts the underlying tissue and drapes the skin over it, removing the excess skin. There are the so-called less-invasive facelifts – the mini lifts – although reports suggest these don't last as long. Whatever type of facelift you have, it will drop over time.

Facelifts

Liposuction

Liposuction is not a method of overall weight loss; it reshapes specific areas. It works on stubborn areas of fat, such as saddle bags, when no amount of dieting or exercise can get rid of them. But lipo is limited to subcutaneous fat and can't be used to remove the dangerous intra-abdominal fat around your middle. And the sad but true fact is that it works better on younger bodies with good skin elasticity. Post-menopause, especially, the results can be less than perfect.

If you've exhausted all other options and opt for hitting the big league, you must do your homework. Find a surgeon with good surgical training and plenty of experience. Don't be swayed by the doctor's charm or the sales patter of the staff and stick to your guns in your quest for the best. It takes time and energy finding Dr Brilliant but you'll thank yourself in the long run.

Some women develop a fat 'pocket' under the eyes as they age. It can be corrected in a fairly simple procedure in which the surgeon cuts a small incision along the lash line, the fat is removed, and the incision is sealed. Results are generally very good. Dark, sagging under-eye bags are a little trickier to fix. If you compare the face of a young person with that of a 50-year-old, you'll see how the cheek 'fat pads' descend with age and dark circles develop under the eyes where the tissue has gone, giving a hollow look. To correct this, the surgeon has to lift the entire cheek fat pad in a mini-facelift. Some doctors fill the hollow area with fat or cosmetic filler.

Got eye baggage?

Sculpture class

The big new thing is facial sculpting. As we age we lose fat from the face. Facelifts can lift dropped cheek pads and reduce excess skin but they can't add volume. Now there's a range of synthetic products that achieve this. Some stimulate the body to produce its own collagen and can be injected into any facial area that needs volume; others are injected at the deepest level – next to the bone itself – to help define a jawline or build up cheekbones. These fillers are also used to fill in the hollow under the eye and just under the eyebrow to help lift the upper lid and reduce drooping.

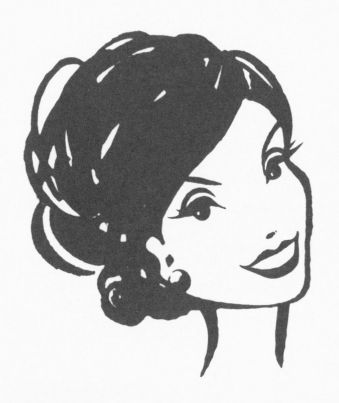

One of the easiest ways a woman in her 50s can lift her look is to invest in professional tooth whitening. You don't have to go over the top and look like you've just stepped off a Hollywood set; a few shades whiter will do. To remove years of coffee, Coca-Cola, smoking and red-wine stains, see your cosmetic dentist for custom bleaching. This can be done over a week or two at home with a special mouth guard and bleaching gel, or – more expensively – as part of an in-rooms procedure with bleaching gel applied under a laser.

One of the best cosmetic treatments

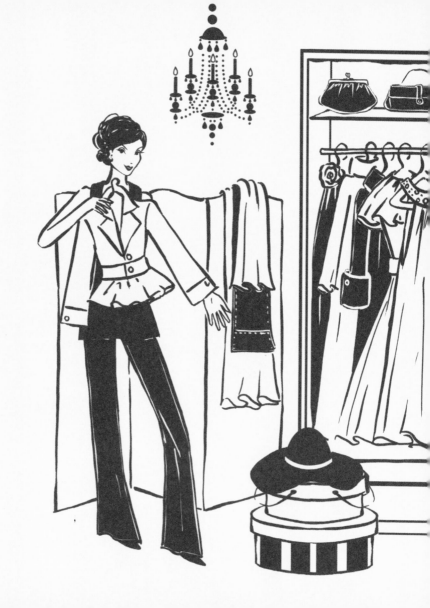

Wardrobe

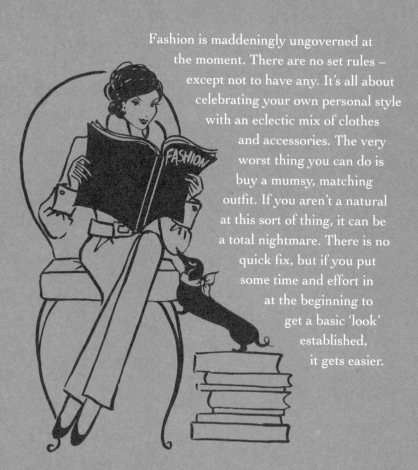

Fashion is maddeningly ungoverned at the moment. There are no set rules – except not to have any. It's all about celebrating your own personal style with an eclectic mix of clothes and accessories. The very worst thing you can do is buy a mumsy, matching outfit. If you aren't a natural at this sort of thing, it can be a total nightmare. There is no quick fix, but if you put some time and effort in at the beginning to get a basic 'look' established, it gets easier.

'Steal' their style

Do some research. Trawl through the various labels in the better department stores. Take in a few hip boutiques. Look at the window displays and make mental notes of what goes with what. Ask the assistant for suggestions and advice. For inspiration have a look at the fashion spreads in the latest magazines. Watch your favourite stars on TV. Don't be above taking note of what other people are wearing as you walk down the street (and ask them where they bought their outfit, if you're brave). Once you have some ideas to start with, you can start developing your own.

EXPERT TIP

If there is a fashion brand that suits you, keep going back to it. This way you can be confident that the pieces will always go together.

Fashion rules for 50-plus

Casual looks younger than formal

★

Don't try to be perfectly turned out

★

Fight the temptation to be overdressed – it's ageing

★

You mustn't look as if you've tried too hard

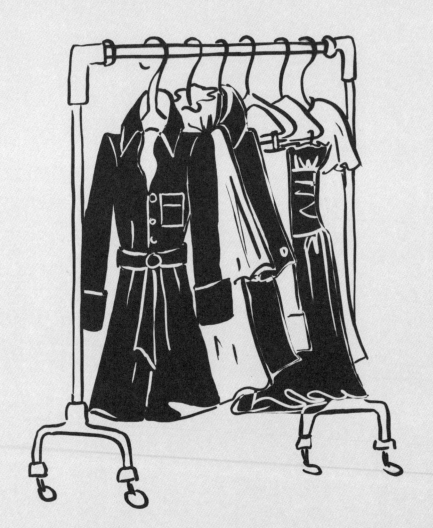

Trends come and go: older women can get away with some 'younger' items as long as they are balanced by good basics

Good basics endure: you can't go wrong with well-cut classics in good materials. The trick is to add a twist with a few stylish items. Best stay away from those that are doomed to be discarded after one season. If you must, source them from the cheaper shops – not the teen departments

Neutrals are your fashion friend: think black and white, beige, tan, silvery grey and navy

Quality fabrics matter: they look better, feel better and survive longer – it's worth the investment

Remember!

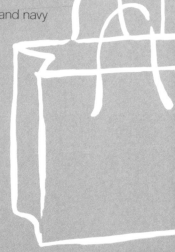

Your essential wardrobe

Tops: cotton T-shirts, black cardigan, cotton V-neck jumper, white blouse or shirt, camisole, cashmere wrap

Bottoms: a couple of pairs of jeans, black tailored pants

Suits: good separates (jacket, pants and skirt) in black or navy

Jackets/coats: denim jacket, trench coat, wool coat

Shoes: black ballet flats, comfy plain sneakers, moccasins, black work pumps, black high heels

Jewellery and accessories: diamond stud/pearl earrings, classic watch, good-quality sunglasses, black work bag, brown everyday bag

MDAL

It's the Mutton Dressed as Lamb debate. How often have you asked when trying something on: 'But do I look like mutton dressed as lamb?' By the time they've hit 50, many women have given up the battle and retreated into fashion frumpiness. But are your old faithfuls really working for you? Or do they just serve to date you, like rings on a tree, back to the decade from which they sprang?

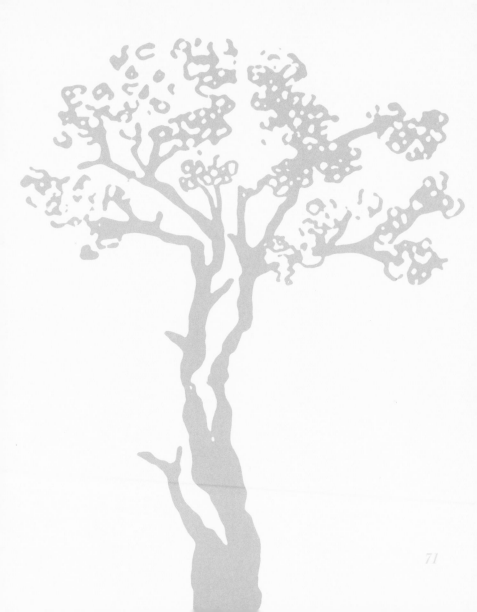

Want to avoid MDAL?

There are no excuses for wearing:

Miniskirts

Hot pants

Ripped or low-slung jeans

Boob tubes

Tie-dyed T-shirts

Ankle bracelets

At the very heart of the MDAL debate is the question of how much to reveal. If you are the kind of girl who harbours an inner lap dancer – don't let her out. Or at least indulge your fantasies in the privacy of your own home. There are a couple of rules:

- Only reveal one bit of flesh at a time. Decide which bits of you look good and make the most of them. If you have a lovely long neck and good shoulders – go strapless. If you have great breasts show a little cleavage. But you should wear neither of these with a short skirt or severely split skirt. If you have great legs wear a short skirt and follow-me-home stiletto heels – but cover up the rest. There is a fine line between flirty and tarty.

- Never wear too tight with too tight – if your skirt or pants are tight, wear a flowing top. If you are wearing a figure-hugging top, wear a more floaty skirt or wide-leg trousers.

Deal-breakers:
bare bits & tight bits

Uh-oh. Are you …

Wearing the same clothes as your partner?

Probably the most extreme reaction to the Mutton Dressed as Lamb debate is the wife-dressed-as-husband response. You know if this is you: polo shirts and khaki shorts in the summer; jeans and baggy jumpers in the winter. If this is your wardrobe you probably look like you're about to set off on a campervan holiday. You need expert help.

Dressing like your mother?

If you find yourself wandering into any one of those shops that specialise in those mother-of-the-bride pastel, synthetic frocks and two pieces, run for your life. This is no way for a 50-year-old to behave. They'll make you look huge. They'll make you look 80. Again, expert help is needed.

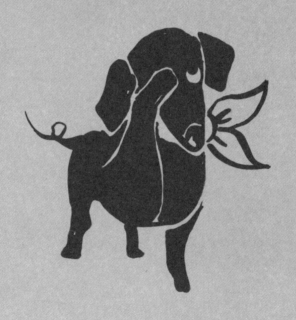

It's time to call in the pros!

Shopping with a friend is pure therapy – and good exercise – but when it comes to fashion advice, you're better off with an independent, professional opinion. Friends tend to be too kind; shop assistants have a vested interest; and partners – well, even if they are among the rare few who don't climb the walls through sheer boredom, they aren't exactly the best judge of women's fashion. They'll either have you in a burka or a naughty maid outfit.

Here's an idea

Ask for a style consultant for your birthday. They'll give you advice that'll last for years. They offer services such as taking you shopping and showing you what clothes you should wear, going through your wardrobe and explaining what items do and don't work. They can advise on colours and make-up. They usually charge by the hour, half day and full day. Look under Image Consultants in the Yellow Pages or online.

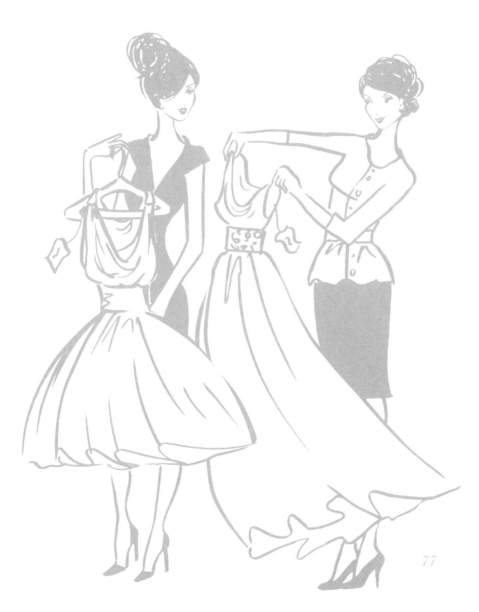

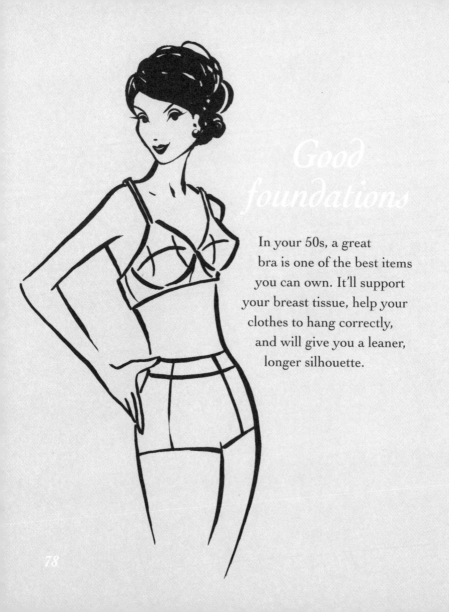

Good foundations

In your 50s, a great bra is one of the best items you can own. It'll support your breast tissue, help your clothes to hang correctly, and will give you a leaner, longer silhouette.

- ★ Have your bra measurements checked every six months in the lingerie section of a department store.

- ★ When shopping for bras, focus on fit rather than on the bra's cup and band size, as different brands fit differently (professional fitting is recommended).

- ★ Avoid that ugly 'back fat' look by adjusting your bra – the middle hook is often the best one.

Bras you must own

The day bra: *also known as the T-shirt bra, it offers seamless support and camouflages nipples*

The sports bra: *essential for protecting delicate breast tissue*

The strapless bra: *great for evening gowns; another option is a multi-tasking bra (the straps can be adjusted to suit different outfits)*

Once, any self-respecting 50-year-old would have been horrified at the idea of wearing jeans. Now the teens of the 1950s are grandmothers and still wearing them.

With so many styles on the market, finding the right pair can be overwhelming. It's up there with finding swimmers – and can be just as depressing. Get it wrong and you look like somebody's mother trying to look hip. Finding the right jeans takes time (don't worry, it's not just you!). Be prepared to try on dozens of pairs before you find the right one; best regard it as a jeans safari – because it could take up several Saturday mornings. But, it's worth it: the right pair of jeans can make you look 10 years younger and kilos lighter. Once you've found *the* pair, celebrate. Then keep going back to the same brand. Here are a few pointers:

Jean genius

Legs Skinny jeans with narrow legs will look too tight and too young, unless you are quite slim. Wide-leg jeans can make you look dumpy if you are short, and blokey if you are big around the middle. The safest option is the straight-leg or the boot-cut.

Fabric A little touch of lycra is a good thing. No stretch, and jeans can be unflattering and uncomfortable. Too much stretch and they look unfashionable and clinging.

Pockets Believe it or not, these are very important. Jeans designers spend time getting it right. Too-small back pockets can make your bum look bigger. Bigger, well-placed pockets can give your bum a visual lift!

If the shoe fits

Have you noticed that more of your friends are complaining about sore feet these days? That's because, as we age, we lose some of the fatty cushioning that protects the balls of our feet. This is the time when bunions and corns make their presence known. Also, any posture problems you may have will increasingly take their toll on your feet.

Thankfully, the shoe industry is now making stylish yet comfy shoes

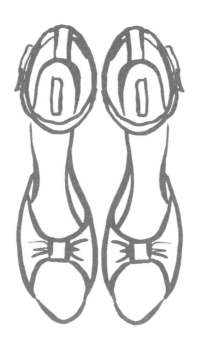

The hallmarks
of a comfortable shoe

★ Generally, the softer and more flexible the shoe, the better (it should bend where your foot naturally bends).

★ Always go for uppers made from a natural material, such as leather, suede or a fabric that allows the foot to 'breathe'.

★ There should be sufficient depth and width at the toes and a short space between the tip of your longest toe and the end of the shoe.

★ The more cushioning the insole has, the longer you'll be able to stand in the shoes.

★ A sole made from rubber provides good shock absorption and is less slippery than leather.

★ A firm heel counter that fits snugly around the back of the foot prevents slipping (and therefore blisters and cramps).

If you hadn't noticed, there is a trend towards bare legs. But, you argue, your legs are flaky, pale and wrinkly – and nothing will get you out of trousers. Well, the good news is that no matter how neglected your pins are, they are one part of the body that responds well to some TLC.

Show some leg!

★ Remove hair – if you are the shaving type, stick with it, but a professional wax is indulgent and longer-lasting.

★ Exfoliate skin – use a loofah in the shower or a gentle scrub.

★ Moisturise twice daily – this will instantly freshen skin; better still, for a golden glow, use one of the new moisturisers that contain a light fake tan.

★ Apply fake tan – a mousse or spray is easiest (and make sure skin is exfoliated and moisturised for best results).

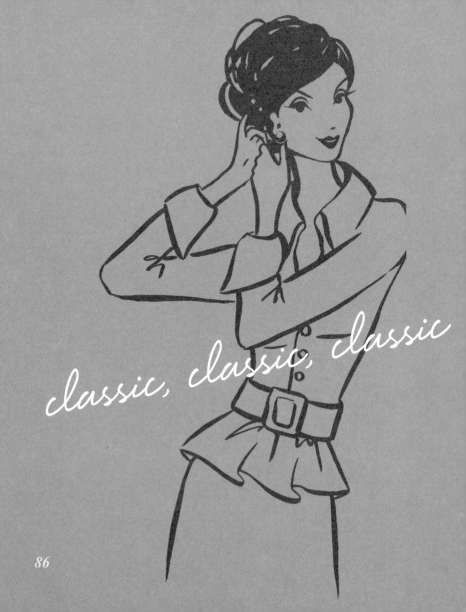

classic, classic, classic

Accessorise

Jewellery, specs and handbags all have their place in high fashion and can instantly update your look. For the 50-something woman, it's all about classic, classic, classic (but this doesn't have to mean expensive!). Nothing ages you faster than frumpy, cheap-looking or damaged accessories.

Jewellery

For jewellery, the current trend is for white gold, platinum and silver with lots of sparkly things – diamonds if your name is Hilton or Beckham, otherwise, zirconias. 'Less is more' is your mantra. The best thing about today's look is that it can be cheap to do; vintage stores and chain-stores are treasure troves.

Glasses

When it comes to specs, please skip the 'old lady' glasses in favour of modern frames. It's amazing how something so small can say so much about your personality. The eyewear industry is big business, producing vast ranges of shapes and styles. Even the major fashion designers such as Prada, Gucci, Chanel and Dior are in on the act. Spend some time choosing your next pair (perhaps invest in a work pair and a weekend pair). Don't buy anything that makes you look like a nerd, a nun or a nanna. And get a second opinion.

Handbags

Barely a week passes without yet another designer bag making the news. But there's no need for logos and expensive price tags. One good-quality bag in natural-toned leather will multi-task very efficiently. *Note:* we have a tendency to stuff our bags with a million things 'just in case' and then carry them over one shoulder. This can cause posture problems, muscle stiffness, tension, pain and headaches. Swap shoulders now and then and edit your bag contents.

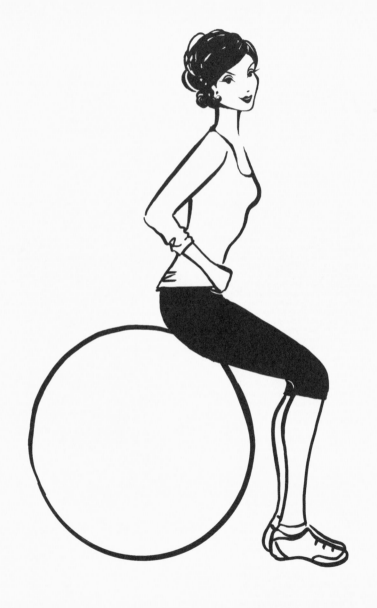

Body

Once it was considered normal for a woman in her 50s to weigh more than she did in her 30s. Now doctors are saying this is wrong. We should weigh the same. The trouble is that middle-age spread creeps up, a kilo or so each year, every year.

Why middle-age spread is oh so bad

By the time you are 50 there is no option but to get serious about your body, diet and exercise regimen (or lack thereof). Now is the time to put in solid work to set you up for the coming decades. No one says it's easy; staying healthy requires constant effort. But the rewards are immense. Yes, you want to look good, but a better long-term approach is to be *healthy*.

We've known for a long time that fat around your middle is especially bad for your health, making you more prone to diabetes, heart disease, stroke and some cancers. Scientists now think middle area fat blocks the body's signalling mechanism for controlling insulin. The system hiccups along, producing too much sugar and then too much insulin. As well as leading to diabetes, an over-production of insulin is thought to cause chronic low level inflammation throughout the body and play a role in hardening of the arteries and heart disease. High insulin levels are also thought to promote the growth of some cancer cells.

Some facts about fat

Losing weight and staying slim is not just about looking good. Obesity is more dangerous than smoking and can shorten your life by as much as 13 years. It contributes to about 10 per cent of cancers in non-smokers and it can increase the risk of heart disease by as much as 2.4 times (from the *Foresight* report written by 250 of the world's top scientists). To make matters worse, another study – conducted in Australia and reported in the *British Medical Journal* – shows that obesity in middle age increases your risk of dementia in old age.

During and just after menopause, losing weight becomes almost impossible. About two-thirds of women will put on weight during this time (typically between five and 10 kilos). Weight comes on gradually, and tends to accumulate around the middle, because of hormones. Hormones have a direct impact on appetite, metabolism and fat storage. Some people develop insulin resistance – a condition where the body stores fat, rather than burning kilojoules.

Menopause and weight gain

Sleep and weight gain

It's been shown that a lack of sleep increases the levels of a hunger hormone and decreases levels of a hormone that makes you feel full. The effects may lead to overeating and weight gain. Scientists have found that people who are chronically sleep-deprived are also overweight. Researchers suggest getting enough sleep might be a critical component of weight control and one day doctors might be recommending to dieters that they 'sleep it off' as well as cut the kilojoules and increase exercise.

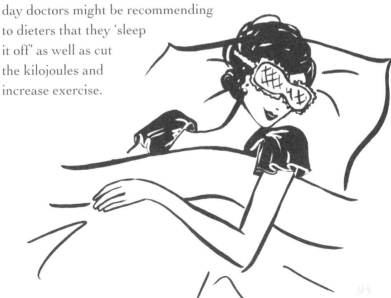

Action!

Regular exercise is one of the best answers to weight gain and stiffness. Everyone who is healthy can exercise. Even if you've hardly run a step since you left the school playground, there's nothing to stop you getting into it in middle age. The secret to staying the distance is to go at your own pace. There are three very important factors to consider:

Weights

From our early 30s we lose about one per cent of muscle mass every year. Muscle means strength, and this is important for balance and avoiding osteoporosis. But muscle also governs our metabolism. Put simply, the more muscle we have, the higher our metabolic rate. The higher our metabolic rate, the easier it is to stay slim. So make sure your exercise regimen includes some light weight training. The good news is that even if you have already lost quite a bit of muscle, it's never too late to start building it up again.

Cardio

One of the best things about walking and running is that they are cheap. All you need is a well-fitting pair of running shoes and a safe, pleasant spot. Aim to work up a sweat for between 30 and 40 minutes about three times a week. Start by walking as briskly as you can for as long as you can. Enjoy the views. Smile at passers-by. Gradually increase the time period and the pace. Only go at the rate at which you feel comfortable. Keep reminding yourself that you are helping your bones rebuild, you are losing fat, and your heart is thanking you for it.

Stretching

Staying flexible is essential for your balance, your posture and for avoiding injury. Simple stretches will do the trick, but yoga and Pilates have huge followings for a very good reason – the professionally taught poses go hand-in-hand with healthy breathing techniques and a very addictive mind calming and clearing effect.

The best 50-something workout

This is the regimen that is recommended as
being optimal for this age group, but, if it seems
too difficult to squeeze into your schedule,
don't forget: *any* activity is good for you.

★ A 20- to 40-minute brisk walk, slow jog or aerobics
class three to five times a week at an intensity that
enables you to answer a question but not chat.

★ Half an hour of weight training twice a week.

Other options

So you hate the gym, resent running and can't see
the point in Pilates? Find a sport or activity that you
enjoy. There's the conventional – cycling, tennis,
swimming, golf, netball, hockey and bushwalking;
and the unconventional – borrow your daughter's
surfboard, give yoga a go, or...

Fling yourself into Flamenco
dancing. It's great for toning legs
and defining waists. Then book
a holiday in Spain.

★

Go back to your girlhood
dreams and go horse-riding.
There's nothing like it for
developing a beautiful bum!

★

Learn kickboxing. It's great for fat
burning, endurance and flexibility. And
it helps you learn to defend yourself.

★

Take up tai chi. It's a low-impact
exercise, increases joint mobility and
is fabulous for relaxation.

★

Take up serious walking. Manage
weight, blood pressure and elevate
your mood with regular hikes.
Then book a walking holiday.

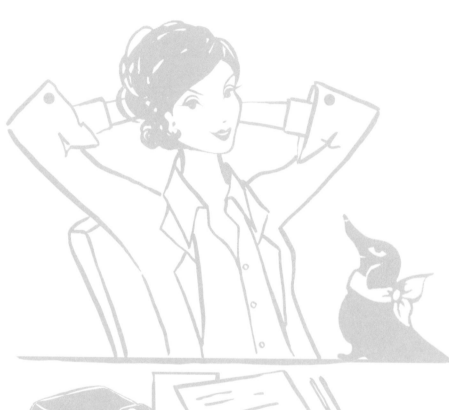

Your 50s is the time to tackle your posture – you really don't want to be a stooping 60-year-old! Losing strength in your core muscles – that run from your pelvis up to your neck – can alter the way you stand and lead to a pot belly. Gradually, you also start to develop rounded shoulders and the classic rounded spine of old age. If you spend your working life hunched over a computer, it's all the worse. A good idea is to see a musculo-skeletal expert (such as a physiotherapist). They'll work on your back, chest and neck muscles to stretch and strengthen them in all the right places. Your private medical insurer may cover some of the costs.

Posture

Simple posture correctors

When you stand, be conscious of clenching your buttocks and pushing forward your pelvic bones. When working at the computer, get up every hour or so, and stretch everything back in the opposite direction. Clasp your hands behind your back and pull your shoulder blades together – feel your chest muscles stretch outwards.

The chest stretch

Stand in an open doorway. Place your hands level with your shoulders on the door frame. Your elbows should also be resting on the door frame. Inhale and, on the exhale, step forward a half step; stay breathing evenly for 20 to 30 seconds. Inhale and, as you exhale, bring the leg back again. Repeat, stepping forward with your other leg.

When working at the computer, get up every hour or so

The back straightener

Take a bath towel, fold it lengthwise and then roll it up to make a sausage. Lie on the floor looking up at the ceiling. Place the rolled-up towel under your back, vertically along your spine, between the shoulder blades and down to about your waist. Feel your body weight pull the chest muscles so that they open out and stretch. Stay there for 10 minutes. Then place the towel horizontally under your back – so that it follows your bra strap – and feel your spine return to a normal position.

You are what you eat

It's time to look at what you're eating. The right foods will not only keep you healthy, but will also help you deal with menopause, boost your energy and improve your looks. It's all about common sense and moderation. Certainly you can't eat as much as you did 20 years ago, but there's no need for severe dieting and deprivation. Choose foods that taste good and do you good, and you'll be set – include wholegrains, lean protein, a colourful array of fresh fruits and vegetables, low-fat dairy and 'good' fats.

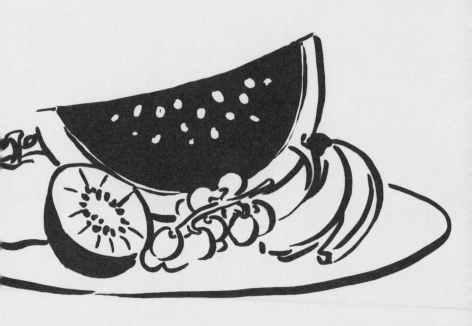

The youth diet

Want to have that youthful glow? Experts recommend a diet that includes low-GI oatmeal, antioxidant-rich berries, green vegetables (such as broccoli), 'good' oils (avocado, nuts, olive oil), omega-3-packed fish (salmon is ideal) and lots of water. Cut down on dehydrating alcohol and caffeine, carcinogenic fried foods and, most of all, cell-damaging sugar.

Oil and water do mix

One of the best things you can do for your brain and body health is to ditch the extreme no-oil or low-fat fad. You'll look and feel better if you eat fat (but continue to avoid saturated fats, found in junk food). Water is another essential – banish tiredness, irritability and headaches with the recommended daily dose of eight glasses.

Having a couple of alcoholic drinks a day can slow bone loss in post-menopausal women. It is also thought to help ward against heart attacks – when taken in moderation. But alcohol has also long been known to increase the risk of breast cancer. This increases with the amount of alcohol consumed. One recent study of 70,000 women showed that three drinks a day was the equivalent risk level as smoking a packet of cigarettes a day. There is no difference between the types of drink. The risk factor is the alcohol itself.

Dieting

Diets come and go, but there is no magic pill
for weight loss. Gaining and losing weight is all
about the little habits you've developed. Every
time you replace a bad habit with a good one, it
is a step in the right direction.

- We often use food as a reward. Try to be aware of when and why you are eating. Use something else as a reward or comfort.

- Stay within your kilojoule allowance and you'll lose weight. If you drop 400 kilojoules from your daily diet, you should lose about 1 kilogram a week.

- Adding exercise to the equation can boost your ability to lose weight; it helps to increase your metabolic rate, even after you've stopped working out.

- Eat smaller portions, and forget what your mother taught you about finishing everything.

- Make a shopping list and don't shop when hungry. If it's in the pantry, you're more likely to be tempted to eat it.

- Be patient; you have to be in it for life. Be warned: go back to your old habits and you'll go back to your old weight.

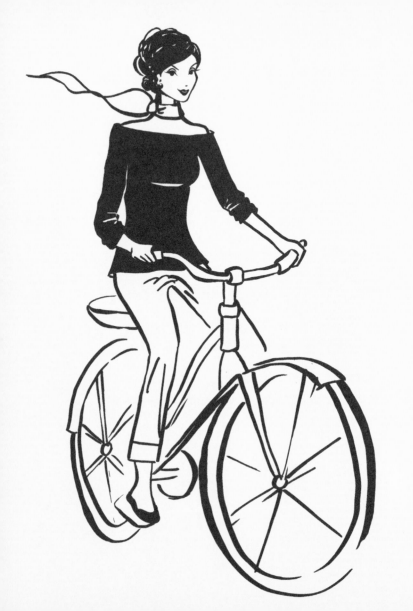

Health

Your 50s is the time to take stock of your health. If you are still smoking and drinking the way you did in your 20s, you have some serious choices to make. What you do now can set the scene for the rest of your life.

Non-negotiable health checks for your 50s

Bowel cancer (colorectal cancer): you should have a Faecal Occult Blood Test (FOBT) at least every two years.

Breast cancer: you should have a mammogram every two years.

Cervical cancer: all women who have had sex and have not had a hysterectomy should have a pap smear every two years.

Coronary disease: you should have a cholesterol and triglycerides blood test every five years.

Dental health: have regular check-ups.

Diabetes: if you are at risk of Type 2 diabetes – such as by having high blood pressure and being overweight – you should have a fasting blood sugar level test every three years.

Eye test – glaucoma/sight degeneration: women over 50 should have their eyes tested every five years.

Obesity: have your BMI – Body Mass Index – checked. You should do this about every two years or, if you are overweight, every 12 months.

Osteoporosis: about the time of menopause, all women should have a bone mineral density test. This is even more important if you have increased risk through early menopause, having a small frame, being a smoker or an excessive coffee drinker.

Skin cancer – melanoma: everybody should check their skin regularly – at least every three months. You should see your doctor every 12 months and they can direct you to a specialist if needed.

Vascular disease: you should have your blood pressure measurement taken every year.

Of course, if you have a family history or other increased risk factors for any of these conditions, your doctor will probably recommend more frequent screening.

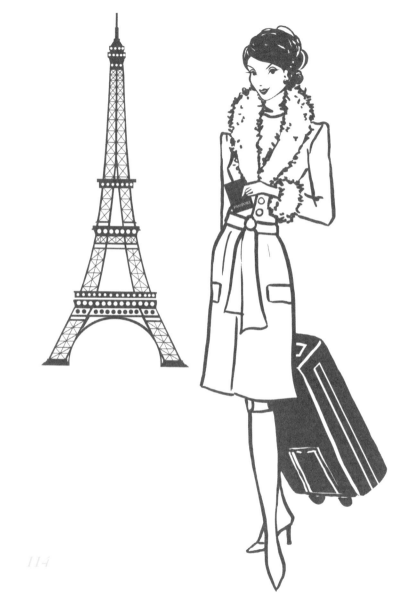

There's no getting away from it and by your 50s you'll be experiencing signs of the 'change' (if you haven't already been through it all). During and immediately after menopause you will see a difference in your mood, muscle tone and metabolism. There is plenty you can do to minimise the impact of menopause. Just look at the thousands of women who survive it looking better than ever.

Menopause

Hot, hot, hot!

Current thinking is that hot flushes occur because lowering oestrogen levels affect the action of the hypothalamus – the region of the brain that controls body temperature. No one really knows why some women are affected worse than others. It's probably partly genetic. Overweight women often fare better because fatty tissue encourages higher oestrogen levels; smokers are more likely to suffer from hot flushes. A few other points:

- Some women sail through menopause without noticing a hot flush; others have to battle them for as long as 10 years.

- Some days and nights seem to be worse than others – this is because oestrogen levels rise and fall as the ovaries cease production.

- HRT can help but, these days, doctors prescribe the lowest possible dose for the shortest possible time. Some doctors prescribe particular anti-depressants, and certain blood-pressure medication has also been shown to help.

* Phytoestrogens – plant chemicals that mimic the action of oestrogen – can help. These include soy milk, tofu, soy flour, lentils, chickpeas, pumpkin and linseed.

* There are concerns about over-the-counter 'natural' hormones because they are not regulated and production is not subject to the same rigorous standards of the mainstream pharmaceutical industry.

5 natural ways to tackle menopause

1 Exercise regularly
2 Take up meditation, tai chi or yoga
3 Add soy-based foods to your diet (and improve the rest of your eating)
4 Dress in natural fibres (cotton, linen, silk), and use layering
5 Sleep in a cool, well-ventilated room

No bones about it

In your 50s, declining oestrogen levels will speed up the rate at which your bones lose calcium, putting you at risk of osteoporosis. Our bones are alive and they grow and change as we do; their health depends on what we eat and how active we are. Every day, your body rebuilds the cells in your bones. This cycle helps repair the tiny fractures and injuries the body suffers daily. The vertebrae in the spine, the hip bones and wrists are the areas that osteoporosis affects the most.

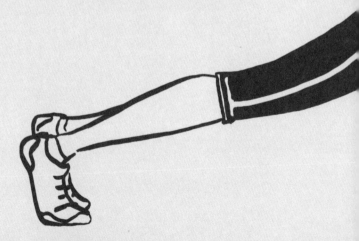

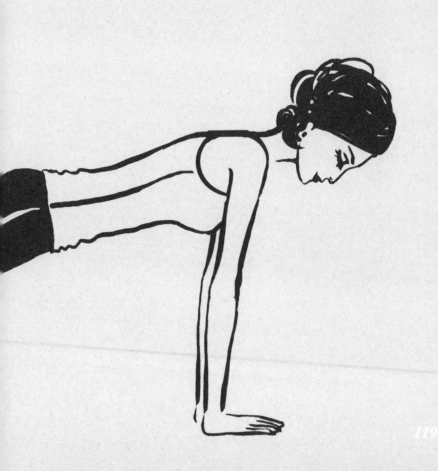

4 things you can do

1 **Take a calcium supplement:** 500 milligrams in the morning; 500 milligrams at night taken with 600 milligrams magnesium

2 **Eat calcium-rich foods:** natural yoghurt, cheese, milk, broccoli and tofu

3 **Cut down on alcohol:** too much reduces the absorption of vitamin D

4 **Do weight-bearing exercise:** running, brisk walking, dancing, tennis or netball are good options. Each time your foot hits the ground you apply stress to your bones; the higher the impact, the greater the benefit to your bones. Note that non-gravity workouts such as swimming and bike riding are good for heart health, but don't build bones.

A note on calcium

The recommended dietary intake of calcium for women is 1000 to 1300 milligrams every day. Most of us are unlikely to achieve this through our diet alone, so supplements can be a useful way of making up the deficit. Taking calcium supplements can slow bone loss, although they do not completely stop it. Find out more about calcium from your GP – and if you haven't already had one, get a bone density scan.

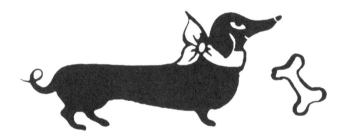

Heart

Heart disease and stroke kill 10 times as many women as breast cancer. In fact, they kill more women than all the cancers combined. Heart disease is the number-one killer, and stroke is the third biggest cause of death in women. More women die from heart disease and stroke than men, yet most of us do not realise we are at risk.

Be prepared

Eighty per cent of strokes are associated with blockages of the arteries in the neck, and are preventable. Some risks you can't do much about . . .

※ being over 55

※ having a family history of stroke

※ being an atrial fibrillation sufferer

But others are lifestyle related . . .

※ high blood pressure

※ high cholesterol

※ atherosclerosis (hardening of the arteries)

※ smoking

※ heavy drinking

※ diabetes

※ not exercising

※ taking Hormone Replacement Therapy (HRT)

※ being overweight

- ☀ sudden numbness or weakness of the face, arm or leg, especially on one side of the body

- ☀ sudden confusion, trouble speaking or understanding

- ☀ sudden trouble seeing in one or both eyes

- ☀ sudden trouble walking, dizziness, loss of balance or coordination

- ☀ sudden severe headache with no known cause

The warning signs

of stroke . . .

The turning-back-the-clock study

Researchers at Yale University have shown that people who eat well and exercise can substantially reduce their risk for cardiovascular disease and death even if they are in their 50s. Consuming at least five fruits and vegetables daily, exercising for at least two and a half hours a week, maintaining a healthy weight and not smoking can lessen your chances of heart trouble by 35 per cent, and your risk of dying by 40 per cent. The Yale team was concerned that some people in middle age do not make lifestyle changes because they think the damage is already done. However, the project showed the chances of dying or having a heart attack were reduced by a third after just four years of living a healthy lifestyle.

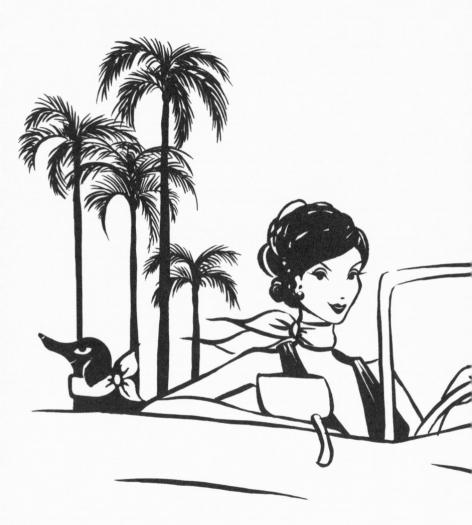

Living

Live it up

Every decade brings change, but it's in their 50s
that many people start a whole new chapter of their
lives. The kids have left home, financially we're more
resilient and perhaps this is the time we start to see that
our years upon this earth are finite.

By contrast, some people have
little choice and are starting
out after a divorce or a job
loss. Regeneration in your
50s can literally be life-
changing, if you work
out what you want
and then plan.

Mid-life brain shift

So, you're in your early 50s and you've suddenly realised that you're wearing the trousers in your partnership? Or you're powering up the corporate ladder? You are not alone.

Ever since you were a little girl your brain has been washed in a sea of female hormones geared to making you reproduce and help the survival of the human species. Of course, there was oestrogen, the hormone that underpins fertility and sexuality. But every time you showed sexual love for your partner or motherly love for your children, you were rewarded with a wave of oxytocin to persuade you to do it all over again.

However, once a woman gets to the menopausal years, the levels of oestrogen and oxytocin decline. In many women, levels of male hormones such as testosterone take over. It makes us more assertive. We are less interested in putting others before ourselves, and we're not afraid to say so.

But, how to 'find' yourself?

After decades of giving to others, it's time to give back to yourself. Channel your restlessness and greater free time into taking care of your physical, mental and spiritual self. This can involve some very simple actions, yet (to begin with) they may be surprisingly hard after so many years of personal neglect. To begin with, set aside an hour a day for yourself. At the same time each day, choose a quiet space and simply sit in stillness, or write whatever comes into your head in a journal. There's no pressure. This is a common tool for allowing the day's 'baggage' to flow in and out of your mind, eventually being replaced with real creative thoughts about what you want to do with your time and your talents.

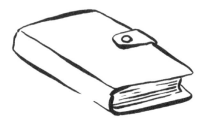

Three simple life-changers

Practise meditation: you don't have to sit alone; it simply means focusing your mind on a particular situation, consciously considering your choices, and making a decision as to how to handle it. It's an exercise and, like any other, you'll become better at it as you flex your brain muscle.

Learn to breathe: it's surprising how many women don't breathe properly. A few times a day, stop and check to make sure you're not breathing shallowly and quickly. Mental clarity and calmness will follow from deep breathing and correct posture.

Keep a journal: you don't have to be a good writer. Put pen to paper and let the thoughts come out, nonsense or otherwise. You'll be amazed at how liberating and healing it can be.

Reinventions can be as small as a new hair cut or joining a weight loss group or as big as retraining for a new job, building a house or travelling overseas. Start by making a plan for your life. Draw up headings such as 'home', 'work', 'personal', 'money', 'relationships'. Look at what is working in your life, and what's not.

Make a wish-list, then refine it. Put down your goals, large and small. Prioritise what's important to you. Then work out the steps you need to achieve them. Don't get too bogged down in the detail. When you reach this point you just have to take a deep breath and jump in.

Achieving our ambitions can help us feel better about ourselves, liven up our lives and make sense of the world. And it doesn't have to interfere with our marriage, work life or relationships with children and friends. Being fulfilled makes us better to be around.

Channel the energy

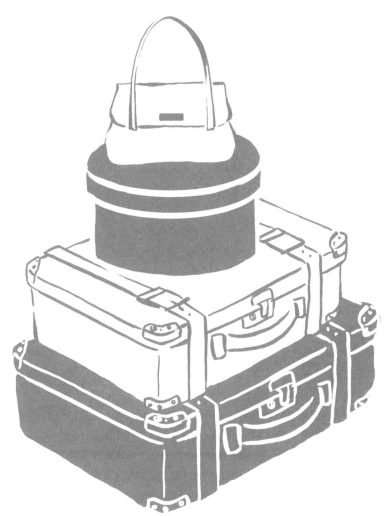

Find a passion and go for it

Research your family history

Develop a talent, such as cooking

Join a political party

Take up a new sport and compete

Write letters on issues to your local newspaper

Learn a musical instrument or a new language

Go travelling – backpack or five-star

Take an adult education class

Build your dream house in the country

It's not all about you!

Adding a new dimension to your life doesn't have to cost money. Helping others is deeply rewarding. It can also help you expand your social network. There are hundreds of positions listed on Volunteering Australia's website. Here are a tiny few:

Tour guide or museum guide

★

RSPCA clerical assistant, fundraiser, event organiser

★

Nursery seedlings planting

★

Fostering native animals

★

Wetlands conservation volunteer

★

Court supporter

★

Bookshop assistant

★

Emergency services radio operator

★

Rescue boat crew

★

First Aid officer

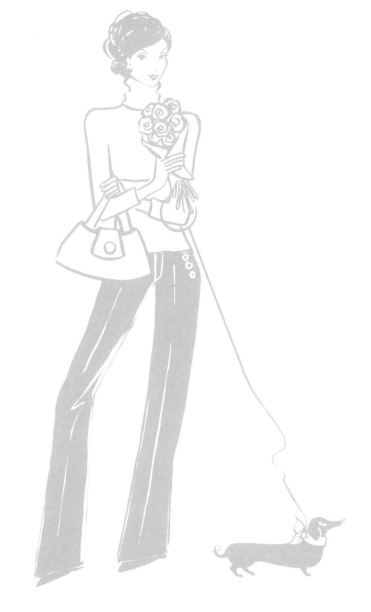

It's up to you. Ignore those people who airily tell you that you should embrace old age and, worse still, those who would rather you slid off quietly into a corner and didn't make a fuss. As long as we live in an ageist world in which women are judged by how old they are and look, and at a time when we have to earn a quid well into our 60s, we can and should say and do anything we deem necessary. When women lie about their age, it's often because they want the world to see that they are still a valuable member of the community and that they count for something. Do remember, however, that 50 isn't what it used to be. After all, Madonna is 50.

Should you lie about your age?

Mid-life crisis, me?

The middle-aged businessman who runs off with his secretary is a cliché. These days it's as likely to be the working 50-something woman who is tempted by an office fling. After 20 or 30 years of marriage, love can grow stale and the prospect of a new love can stave off the feelings of inevitable mortality. It's easy to get swept away – especially if sex with someone new is on the horizon and you've been faithful all your married life. For the middle-aged 'virgin', admiration from someone new can be a head spinner. But don't be undone by your vanity. If you find you are in the grip of an overwhelming crush, take a look at what's motivating you. Although we like to think we're just overtaken by love, it's not that simple – or dramatic. These feelings don't just arrive, we create them. Try to analyse them. What is it about this person? What is it about your partner? How much do you have to lose? What will you gain?

Be a doer, not a dreamer. It's easy to let life slip by. But if you stop every now and then, take stock, and work out solid goals for the next part of your life, you'll find that you can pack so much in. More importantly, you can do the things that are important to you. Decide on one action that you can do today, and go for it. See you in your 60s!

Just do it

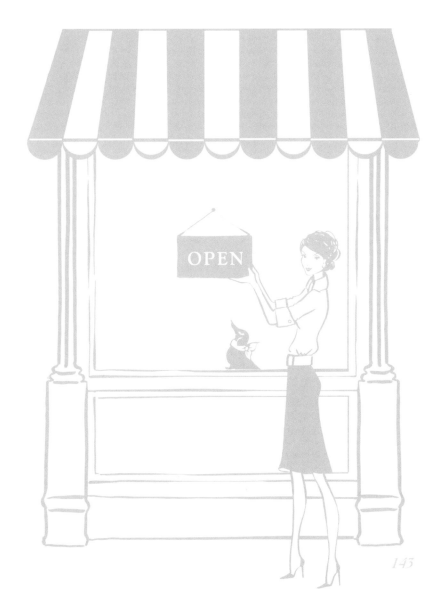

An Ebury Press book
Published by Random House Australia Pty Ltd
Level 3, 100 Pacific Highway, North Sydney, NSW 2060
www.randomhouse.com.au

First published by Ebury Press in 2008

Addresses for companies within the Random House Group can be found at
www.randomhouse.com.au/offices.

National Library of Australia
Cataloguing-in-Publication Entry

    Robson, Pamela.
    Grown-up & gorgeous in your 50s.

    ISBN 978 1 74166 802 5 (pbk.)

    Beauty, Personal.Women – Health and hygiene.
    Middle-aged women – Health and hygiene.

    646.7042

Cover and internal illustrations by Megan Hess
Cover design by Christabella Designs
Internal design by Anna Warren, Warren Ventures Pty Ltd
Additional design by Liz Seymour, Seymour Designs
Printed and bound by Tien Wah Press (PTE), Singapore

Random House Australia uses papers that are natural, renewable and recyclable products and made from wood grown in sustainable forests. The logging and manufacturing processes are expected to conform to the environmental regulations of the country of origin.

10 9 8 7 6 5 4 3 2 1